YOUR KNOWLEDGE HAS VALUE

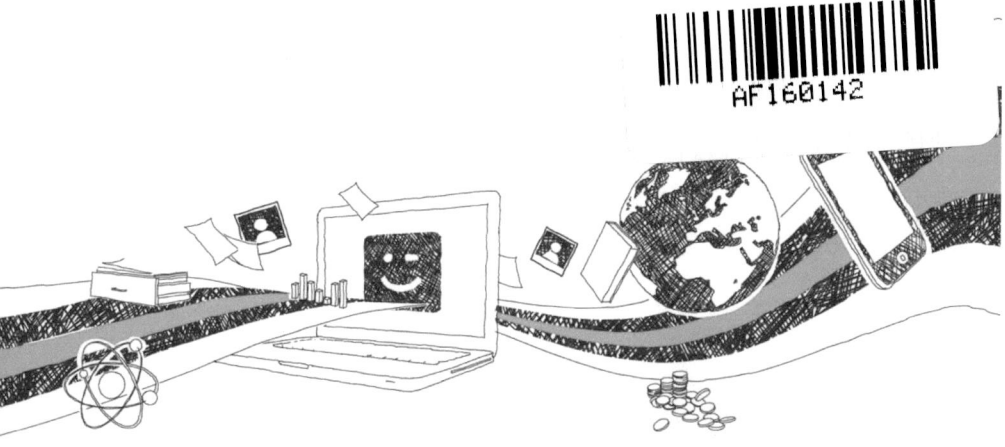

- We will publish your bachelor's and master's thesis, essays and papers

- Your own eBook and book - sold worldwide in all relevant shops

- Earn money with each sale

Upload your text at www.GRIN.com and publish for free

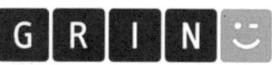

Bibliographic information published by the German National Library:

The German National Library lists this publication in the National Bibliography; detailed bibliographic data are available on the Internet at http://dnb.dnb.de .

This book is copyright material and must not be copied, reproduced, transferred, distributed, leased, licensed or publicly performed or used in any way except as specifically permitted in writing by the publishers, as allowed under the terms and conditions under which it was purchased or as strictly permitted by applicable copyright law. Any unauthorized distribution or use of this text may be a direct infringement of the author s and publisher s rights and those responsible may be liable in law accordingly.

Imprint:

Copyright © 2016 GRIN Verlag, Open Publishing GmbH
Print and binding: Books on Demand GmbH, Norderstedt Germany
ISBN: 9783668575479

This book at GRIN:

http://www.grin.com/en/e-book/381226/dual-diagnosis-of-substance-abuse-and-depression

Patrick Kimuyu

Dual Diagnosis of Substance Abuse and Depression

GRIN - Your knowledge has value

Since its foundation in 1998, GRIN has specialized in publishing academic texts by students, college teachers and other academics as e-book and printed book. The website www.grin.com is an ideal platform for presenting term papers, final papers, scientific essays, dissertations and specialist books.

Visit us on the internet:

http://www.grin.com/

http://www.facebook.com/grincom

http://www.twitter.com/grin_com

MENTAL HEALTH, DUAL DIAGNOSIS OF SUBSTANCE ABUSE AND DEPRESSION

Name: Patrick K. Kimuyu

Substance abuse and co-occurring disorders are seemingly becoming an enormous challenge to health care systems. Substance abuse has become popular, especially among the young people even though its prevalence appears to be a cross-sectional health issue with drug addiction occurring across all ages and gender. On the other hand, mental illnesses are increasing at an alarming rate among the global population; thus, unprecedented burden to healthcare systems and professionals. Ordinarily, the occurrence of a mental health issue such as depression and a substance abuse problem is what is commonly referred to as dual diagnosis or a co-occurring disorder. From a nursing perspective, dual diagnosis does not appear to be a simple task because it deals with handling two problems concurrently: the mental health problem and the substance abuse issue. Saisan, Segal and Smith (2013) remark, "Dealing with substance abuse, alcoholism, or drug addiction is never easy, and it's even more difficult when you're also struggling with mental health problems, but there are treatments that can help" (par. 1). Therefore, a nurse requires extensive understanding on dual diagnosis, so as to provide efficient support and proper treatment to the patient. Moreover, overcoming dual diagnosis requires the nurse to guide the patient in developing efficient self-help strategies for recovery.

Understanding the nature of dual diagnosis involves a comprehensive evaluation of the symptoms of the mental health problem and substance abuse. For instance, in a case where the mental health disorder is depression interacting with substance abuse problem such as alcohol or drug addiction, the two issues requires a comprehensive evaluation prior to the adoption of the appropriate treatment option.

Depression is one of the most common mental health disorders among the global population. It manifests itself through an array of symptoms; thus, different individuals portray different depression symptoms, making it difficult to determine whether an individual is depressed or not. However, there are some common symptoms of depression which can help a nurse to identify the mental health disorder. Ordinarily, depression is determined through the use of a combination of five or more symptoms including loss of pleasure or sadness. Some of the most common symptoms of depression are constant exhaustion, loss of appetite, change of sleep patterns, anger and anxiety. Other significant symptoms of depression include guilt-feeling, pessimism, unable to concentrate in decision making, isolation from other people and suicidal feelings. In most cases, aches in various body parts and pains accompany other depression symptoms (DBSA, n.d).

On the other hand, substance abuse behavior can be identified through the use of different symptoms. Ideally, an array of symptoms is used to rule out drug addiction among the affected individuals. For instance, drug abuse among teenagers is manifested by problems at school such as the reduction of academic performance, physical health issues such as exhaustion and lack of energy, and an abrupt change in social behavior. In some cases, neglected appearance among teenagers and changes in their money spending tendencies serve as some of the principal indicators of substance abuse (Mayo Clinic, 2013).

It is believed that the co-occurring disorders interact synergistically to produce the overall effect observed in co-morbidity patients. In some cases, the presence of untreated mental health issue enhances the severity of the substance abuse problem. However, the advancement of the substance abuse problems causes an increase in the impact of the mental health disorder; thus, causing unprecedented complication. For instance, drug or alcohol abuse has been found to increase mental health disorders, especially with regard to depression.

However, it is worth to understand the basis of the co-occurring disorders and their relationship among individuals. As such, a nurse has to understand which of the co-occurring disorders appears first or which of the two problems influence the onset of the other. Clinical research indicates that, most people with mental health problems tend to be addicted to drugs. However, it is worth noting that, neither substance abuse nor depression or anxiety influence the cause of each other, even though, these two problems are linked. In most cases, symptoms of depression are often self-medicated using drugs or alcohol because they seem to relieve individuals of depression. However, the mental health problem may become worse, owing to the side effects of substance abuse. In such circumstances, the mental health disorder can be viewed to as the cause of substance abuse (Saisan, Segal & Smith, 2013).

On the other hand, the risk of mental health disorders has been found to be increased by substance abuse. Ordinarily, interplay of different factors such as genetic, social and environmental factors is believed to be the cause of mental health disorders, but substance abuse enhances the strength of the underlying risk factors to establish the mental health disorder (Fleming & Hanson, 2013). In such a case, substance abuse can be viewed to as the cause of the mental health problem because the other underlying risk factors are not manifested during the onset of the mental health problem.

Moreover, the symptoms of most mental health problems, including depression are believed to be worsened by substance abuse. For instance, alcohol or drug abuse among individuals with mental health problems triggers new symptoms or increase the severity of the existing symptoms. In regard to medication, alcohol or drug abuse influences the impact of medication with anti-depressants, mood stabilizers and anti-anxiety pills. In general, substance abuse reduces the efficacy of medication administered to address mental health disorders such as depression (Saisan, Segal & Smith, 2013). Therefore, substance abuse interferes with the management of mental health problems, leading to unprecedented complications among the affected individuals.

In regard to the treatment of dual diagnosis, management of dual diagnosis aims at treating the symptoms of the co-occurring disorders. For instance, treatment for individuals with substance abuse problem and depression focuses on relieving the symptoms of depression through medical approaches while mitigating the substance abuse issue. Therefore, treatment of mental health illnesses and drug addiction should be addressed all together for the realization of remarkable recovery (Fleming & Hanson, 2013). Despite the complexity of the treatment of dual diagnosis, efficient therapeutic approaches help to eliminate the problems; thus, helping the affected individuals to reclaim their lives.

In general, treatment of dual diagnosis involves different approaches, especially with regard to the mental health problem and substance abuse involved. Currently, health care professionals are addressing the issue of co-occurring disorders from what is commonly referred to as effective integrated treatment. Ideally, patients with co-occurring disorders require an elaborate treatment approach to address the problems involved. This is so because; addressing a single issue does not help the patient to recover from the afflictions caused by the co-occurring disorders. Research indicates, "If both are recognized, the individual may bounce back and forth between services for mental illness and those for substance abuse, or they may be refused treatment by each of them. Fragmented and uncoordinated services create a service gap for persons with co-occurring disorders" (Drake, 2003 par. 4). Therefore, effective integrated treatment is the most reliable approach in helping patients with co-occurring disorders to realize absolute recovery. Drake (2003) remarks, "Providing appropriate, integrated services for these consumers will not only allow for their recovery and improved overall health, but can ameliorate the effects their disorders have on their family, friends and society at large" (par. 4).

In practice, effective integrated treatment for dual diagnosis involves same health professionals who work together in one setting in providing dual diagnosis treatment to individuals with substance abuse and mental health problems in a coordinated fashion. Therefore, nurses are supposed to ensure that interventions are coordinated so that individuals with co-occurring disorders receive consistent treatment. As such, they are not supposed to handle mental health disorders and substance abuse are two different issues, but rather as a collective issue. Despite the differences observed between the traditional mental health counseling and substance abuse counseling, nurses should reconcile these two approaches for effective treatment of co-occurring disorders. Moreover, nurses should abandon a moralistic model in treating co-occurring disorders and replace it with an efficient illness model which aims at helping patients to realize recovery from both problems (Drake, 2003).

In general, an integrated treatment program for co-occurring disorders involves several factors, which determine the success of the treatment process with remarkable recovery. Some of the most principal factors include approaching treatment in stages, assertive outreach and motivational interventions.

First, nurses should ensure that the integrated treatment program is designed to suit the needs of the patient; hence, trust must be cultivated between the caregiver and the patient, so as to enhance the patient's motivation towards learning the appropriate skills for controlling the problem. This helps to prevent relapse during the treatment process. The second key factor in the integrated treatment program is that, nurses should establish assertive outreach to engage patients to the program to facilitate monitoring and evaluation of the patient's progress with regard to treatment. Thirdly, in the effective integrated treatment, nurses should adopt motivational interventions through counseling and educating their patients. Moreover, they should offer social support to their patients to help them cope with the challenges in the ambient environment which exerts direct impacts on their social nature, especially with regard to moods and personal choices (Drake, 2003).

However, it is worth noting that, treatment of dual diagnosis encompasses numerous successes and challenges. In regard to effective integrated treatment, a number of aspects in the treatment program help to remove the barrier experienced in addressing dual diagnosis. Sciacca (1997) states, "Dual diagnosis treatment approaches and motivational interviewing interventions represent far-reaching changes for substance abuse treatment and comprehensive services, within both the mental health and substance abuse systems" (p. 47). This is probably so because; the traditional treatment programs of substance abuse and mental health disorders failed to address dual disorders, leading to slow success. Therefore, the effective integrated treatment offers a reliable treatment approach to dual diagnosis with appreciable success.

On the other hand, dual diagnosis encompasses several challenges. One of the most significant challenges involved in the treatment of dual diagnosis is non-compliance to the treatment approaches. NHS (2009) reports, "Service users with a dual diagnosis are more likely to be non-compliant and fail to respond to treatment than people with substance misuse issues or a mental illness" (p. 2). The second challenge associated with the treatment of dual diagnosis is finding the right treatment for patients with dual diagnosis disorders. These disorders involve enormous complexity, especially with regard to their social, physical and psychological nature which influences detection, treatment, assessment and the provision of quality nursing care (NHS, 2009). Besides, the cost involved in the treatment of dual disorders is relatively overwhelming to the local healthcare systems, causing most of the treatment programs unsuccessful.

In regard to therapeutic relationships and treatment interventions with dual diagnosis, therapeutic approaches do not yield success unless they are combined with counseling and other motivational initiatives. For instance, therapeutic treatment of depression with anti-depressants does not eliminate the mental health problem, as long as; the patient is not guided to quit substance abuse. Ordinarily, administration of anti-depressants to an individual with dual diagnosis will suppress the symptoms of depression, but that will not address the underlying risk factors. Therefore, recovery from dual diagnosis requires a combination of therapeutic, especially with regard to medication and psychiatric services, as well as, peer support. Helping individuals recovering from dual diagnosis may include showing the person appropriate self-help support groups where they learn different aspects from their peers with real-life experiences (Saisan, Segal & Smith, 2013).

In the past, evidence based practice in mental health nursing practice was not considered as a significant approach to the treatments and care for patients with mental illnesses. This is probably the reason as to why the introduction of evidence-based practice in nursing has aroused unprecedented controversy. Happell and Fisher (2009) reaffirms, "The introduction of evidence-based practice (EBP) and the hierarchical approach to evidence it engenders within research and evaluation has aroused controversy in the mental health professions" (p. 179). However, different health policy planners are advancing towards making evidence-based practice a reality despite the challenges involved in the approach. Cleary and his colleagues report, "In recent years, efforts have been directed towards making mental health nursing more evidence-based. Making evidence based practice (EBP) a reality in modern health services requires due attention to service planning and management; it is acknowledged that there are many challenges and barriers in implementing EBP" (278).

It is believed that, the adoption of evidence-based practice in mental health nursing will require all psychological interventions to mental health disorders to be evidence-based, and this will serve as a comforting paradox. In other words, all counseling will be evidence-based because, "non-specific effects and investigator allegiance suggest that the most competently administered forms of counseling provided by mental health nurses could be seen as being evidence based, even if there is no direct evidence to support the specific models used" (Paley & Shapiro, 2001, p. 34). Canadian Nurses Association (2013) explains that evidence-based practice will enhance decision-making in the nursing. The significance of evidence informed decision-making is that, "patients depend on nurses to do the best on their behalf; as part of their professional accountability, nurses must continually examine the best way to deliver care" (par. 4). Therefore, it is recommended that education sessions are necessary to assist the mental health nurse's clinical decision making and practice base.

References

Cleary, M. et al. (2005). Making evidence based practice a reality for mental health nursing. *Contemp Nurse.* 20(2):278-89.

CNA (2013). *Evidence-based practice: evidence-informed Decision-making.* retrieved from http://www.nurseone.ca/Default.aspx?portlet=StaticHtmlViewerPortlet&plang=1&ptnme =Evidence-based%20practice%20home

DBSA (n.d.). *Dual diagnosis and recovery.* Retrieved from http://www.dbsalliance.org/site/PageServer?pagename=education_brochures_dual_diagn osis

Drake, R. (2003). *Dual Diagnosis and Integrated Treatment of Mental Illness and Substance Abuse Disorder.* Retrieved from http://www.nami.org/Template.cfm?Section=By_Illness&Template=/TaggedPage/Tagge dPageDisplay.cfm&TPLID=54&ContentID=23049

Fleming, P. & Hanson, G. (2013). *Mental illness: the challenges of dual diagnosis.* Retrieved from http://learn.genetics.utah.edu/content/addiction/issues/mentalillness.html

Happell, B. & Fisher, J. E. (2009). Implications of evidence-based practice for mental health nursing. *Int J Ment Health Nurs.* 18(3):179-85. doi: 10.1111/j.1447-0349.2009.00607.x.

NHS (2009). *Seeing double: meeting the challenge of dual diagnosis.* Retrieved from http://www.nhsconfed.org/Publications/Documents/Seeing_double-briefing.pdf

Paley, G. & Shapiro, D. (2001). Evidence-based psychological interventions in mental health nursing. *Nursing Times,* 97(3): 34. Retrieved from http://www.nursingtimes.net/nursing-practice/clinical-zones/mental-health/evidence-based-psychological-interventions-in-mental-health-nursing/206109.article

Saisan, J., Segal, J. & Smith, M. (2013). *Substance abuse & mental health*. Retrieved from http://www.helpguide.org/mental/dual_diagnosis.htm

Sciacca, K. (1997). Removing barriers: dual diagnosis and motivational interviewing. *Professional Counselor* 12(1): 41-7. Retrieved from http://www.treatment.org/Topics/pdf/SciaccaRemovingBarriers.pdf

1. Mayo Clinic (2013). *Drug addiction*. Retrieved from http://www.mayoclinic.com/health/drug-addiction/DS00183/DSECTION=symptoms
2. Barrett, M., Lewellen, A. & Watkins, T. (2001). *Dual diagnosis: an integrated approach to treatment*. New York, NY: Sage.

YOUR KNOWLEDGE HAS VALUE

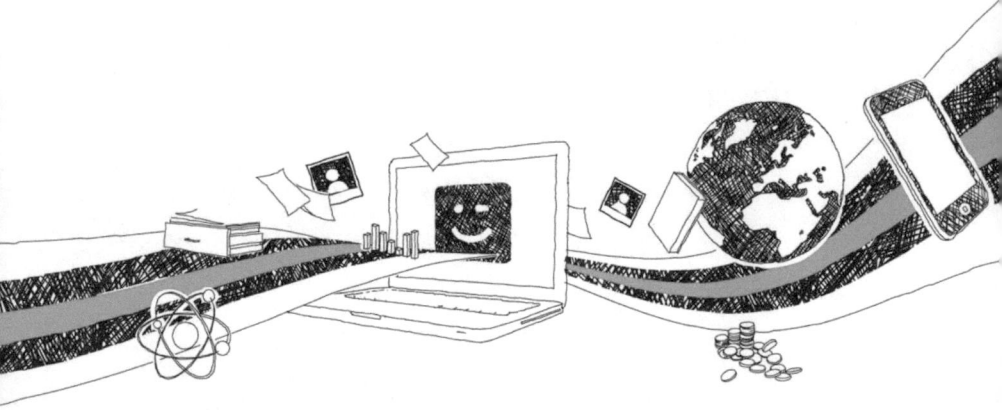

- We will publish your bachelor's and
  master's thesis, essays and papers

- Your own eBook and book -
  sold worldwide in all relevant shops

- Earn money with each sale

Upload your text at www.GRIN.com
and publish for free

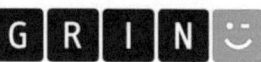